Ten Wild Herbs For Ten Modern Problems

Facing Today's Health Challenges With Holistic Herbal Remedies

By Mary Thibodeau

Disclaimer: This book is not intended as a substitute for the medical advice of your health care practitioner. The reader should regularly consult a physician in matters relating to his/her health and diet, and particularly with respect to any symptoms that may require diagnosis or medical attention.

TABLE OF CONTENTS

Chapter 10

Motherwort for Heart Disease

Conclusion:

Embracing a Natural Choice

The Holistic Approach

Today we face the challenges presented by the lifestyles we have chosen. Our fast paced, ever changing society creates health problems that are not just common, but rampant. Pollution, poor eating habits, excessive work hours, stress and many other modern factors prevalent in western society are continually taking their toll.

Foraging for wild plants and medicinal herbs offers the holistic approach to today's symptoms of a world that is out of balance. Herbs from the wild can help relieve ailments, yes, but they also are part of a getting back to nature approach to living in harmony with the earth and our own bodies.

In this book I have outlined some of the problems facing my own readers and thousands of others with similar issues. I think people are ready to embrace wild plants not only for their medicinal actions, which are largely devoid of harmful side effects, but also for their nutritional value and the lifestyle changes that develop as you learn to take part in the ancient art of wildcrafting herbs.

The act of foraging (or *wildcrafting* as I like to call it) can encompass many healthy habits within itself. When wildcrafting, you are ingesting ultra fresh, highly nutritional food, enjoying a close connection to the earth, and getting in some exercise, sun and fresh air. All these things in turn can lessen the effects of the modern health issues for which we are seeking solutions. Simply by the act of wildcrafting you are creating for yourself a holistic approach to your problem. Using medicinal and wild herbs is a wonderful way to complement your health and wildcrafting the plants yourself brings you closer to true vitality.

Thank you for joining me in learning about the herbs nature has provided for us. Together we will discover how these plants can be used, and how they can benefit our health.

How to Use This Book

These herbs can all be harvested in the wild somewhere on earth and most of them can be found in Europe, Asia and the Americas. But chances are you will not have all of them in your backyard. If you find what looks like any of these herbs in your area, it's important to have a botanist, herbalist or other plant professional make a positive I.D. before you do any harvesting or medicinal dosing. Many of the herbs talked about below have numerous species and look-alikes in the wild. Always verify that you are absolutely sure of the species before picking or using any wild plants.

Luckily, most of the herbs in my book, with the exception of Boswellia, can be cultivated organically at home so you have a fresh source of medicine. To me, the differences between wild and cultivated lie in the freshness and quality. If you are buying a cultivated herb from an online source, that herb may have been sprayed to preserve freshness and harvested years ago. On the other hand, if you are growing herbs organically, in my opinion, that is just as good as wild.

Please take special note of the warnings under certain herbs. These plants have potent properties that can sometimes mix negatively with other medications or increase unwanted side effects. The dosage recommendations listed in each chapter are for a healthy adult. To receive dosage information for children, pregnant women and those compromised by other health factors, seeking the advice of a healthcare practitioner before using herbs is strongly advised.

Chapter 1
St. John's Wort
For Physical and Emotional
Pain

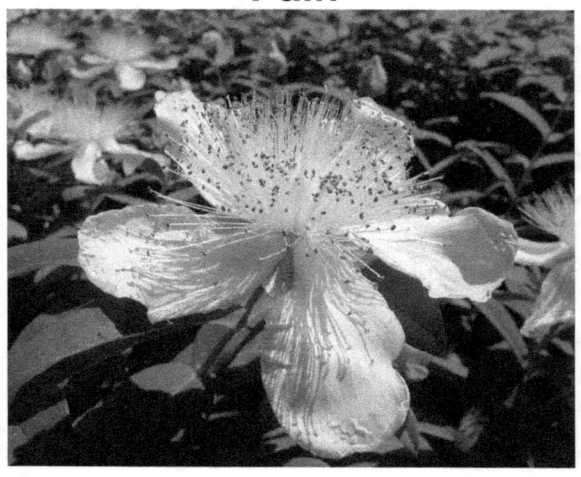

This gorgeous herb with its starlike yellow flowers grows profusely in fields and meadows near my home in Maine. They are particularly prolific in our wild blueberry barrens despite regular pesticide sprays. A native to Europe and Asia, St. John's Wort is now prevalent in the U.S., Canada and Australia. Its name derives from the fact that its first blooms are often seen in Europe and the U.K. right around the birthday of St. John the Baptist, June 24th. Here in

Maine, I usually see the first flowers about two weeks after the 24th.

Its nickname, "Demon Chaser", says it all about Saint John's Wort's ability to ward off emotional and physical pain. Taken internally, it provides two nervous system targeting components: hypericin and hyperforin; which act specifically on chemical messengers in regulating moods. The effects include calming of the nervous system, relief of mild to moderate depression and anxiety, and alleviation of nerve pain.

Externally, St. John's Wort lowers the temperature of the skin and acts as a natural antibiotic making it the perfect herb for dressing wounds and burns. It works directly toward reducing pain caused by inflammation in cases of gout, neuralgia, sciatica, gastritis and arthritis.

WARNING: St. John's Wort should only be taken internally after discussion with your healthcare practitioner. I am not just saying this to cover my butt. If this herb is taken with other medications (especially MAOI inhibitors and other antidepressants), it can cause a condition called serotonin syndrome, which may lead to seizures or death. St. John's Wort on it's own is a potent medicinal herb with many added nutritional benefits and positive side effects. Mixed with other drugs it can dangerously increase the side effects of those prescriptions. St. John's Wort may also cause sun sensitivity in some people, but as a fair skinned person who's outside a lot, I have not noticed this effect. It would be prudent to avoid bright light therapies, tanning beds and excessive outdoor time when taking St. John's Wort internally for a long period.

How to Use St. John's Wort

Internally for Anxiety & Depression

TEA
If you have St. John's Wort in your area that you can harvest, simply cut the top six inches of the plant (including leaves, flowers and stems) and lay them out to dry in a warm, breezy spot out of the sun. If it's not humid, they should dry within a week. Otherwise you can dry them in a gas oven with only the pilot light, and the door slightly open. This

method is faster and the herb should be ready to use in a few days.

Whether you are using your own herb or have bought some online or at a natural foods market, place a handful of the dried herb into a pot of boiling water and turn off the heat. Let infuse for 20 minutes, strain and then drink. 1-3 cups per day is the standard dose.

CAPSULES
To me, having a cup of herbal tea is the best way to take medicine, but taking capsules of the dried herb daily is convenient and effective. You can encapsulate your own by purchasing a simple capsule machine for under $20.00 U.S. dollars or you can buy the supplements online or in a natural foods store. If you do purchase them, I would look for organic sources. The recommended dose for mild to moderate depression is 300 mg taken three times per day.

Externally for Burns, Wounds and Pain

FIRST AID SALVE
Around my house, we call this Magic Salve. It is the remedy for any and all

boo boos. Over the years I have made many different versions and I'm always trying new combinations of herbs. But the recipe below is specifically for burns and pain. You can also buy a St. John's Wort based salve online or in stores but you will save a lot of money by doing it yourself.

Step 1-Make the infused oil. Heat (never boil) 1 cup of dried St. John's Wort herb in 1 cup of olive oil for 20-30 minutes (other oils that work nicely include grape seed oil and almond oil). Then strain well with cheesecloth or a non-bleached coffee filter squeezing out all the oil. Place in a glass jar, colored if you have one.

Step 2-Mix with beeswax. Combine 1 part beeswax with 5 parts St. John's Wort oil. Warm until the beeswax is completely melted into the oil. I use a dedicated Plexiglas measuring cup that can be warmed on the stove, and with the measurements on the side of the glass, it is easy to make the proper ratios. I also have one pan just for melting beeswax.

Step 3-Stir in optional ingredients. I like to put in about 10-20 drops of 100% Pure Lavender Essential Oil for its scent and antibacterial and soothing properties. I also add 3-5 drops of Vitamin E Oil, which acts as a preservative.

Step 4-Pour into your recycled glass or plastic containers. Let cool completely; they will harden up a bit. Then cover and store in a cool dark place.

In the past my family has used this salve (or close variations) for splinters, cuts, bug bites, sunburns, kitchen burns (if you are a serious cook, this should be in your kitchen!), bruises, sore muscles, nerve pain, sprains, cold sores, chapped lips, etc. It's a non-toxic product that is safe for babies and doesn't hurt if it gets in the eyes or mouth accidentally.

Chapter 2
Wild Chamomile
For Inflammation and
Calming

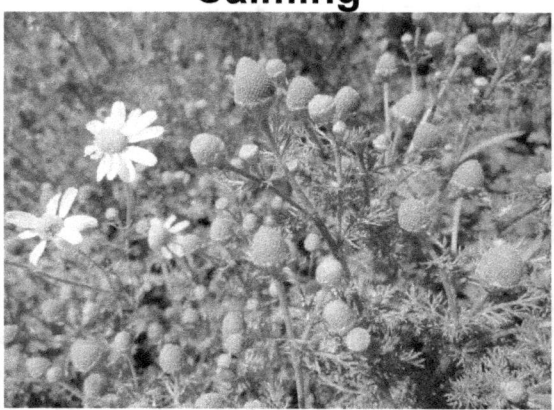

Many people have enjoyed a cup of chamomile tea, though it was probably a cultivated Roman or German Chamomile variety. For inflammation, all types of chamomile are interchangeable, with the wild version being, of course, my favorite. Foraged chamomile is more closely related to the German strain except it does not produce petals on its flowers. If you don't have a place to wildcraft this herb, feel free to substitute the cultivated varieties.

Found across Eurasia, North Africa, Australia and the Americas, you have probably at some point in your life stepped on Wild Chamomile. It is low growing and, because it does not have flashy flowers, it tends to blend in with fields and grass.

Chamomile has for centuries enjoyed the reputation of being a soothing remedy for numerous ailments and medical studies now back up its many abilities. As a powerful yet gentle nervine, chamomile relaxes and tones the nervous system, calms a nervous stomach, aids in sleep disorders, relieves cramps, reduces fevers and acts as a mild diuretic. Safe for children, the elderly and those who are sick, this herb causes anti-inflammatory action in cases of gout, eczema, gastritis, rashes, hemorrhoids, allergies, wounds, burns, IBS and ulcerative colitis. Many of these inflammatory conditions have at their root, stress. Chamomile not only helps relieve the symptoms, but also works on the stress behind the disease.

When harvesting Wild Chamomile, simply cut the flowering tops and dry. Store in a glass jar out of the light.

WARNING: Because Chamomile in large doses may induce uterine contractions, it is not recommended for pregnant women.

How To Use Chamomile

Internally as an Anti-inflammatory and Nerve Tonic

While chamomile can certainly be taken as a capsulized daily supplement, I recommend having at least one cup of the tea every day to relieve inflammation and stress. The art of making the tea and the time spent relaxing with a warm, soothing drink, add extra benefits for an over-taxed body.

TEA
You may use the same instructions for making tea with a wildcrafted herb found in the previous chapter, or you can easily buy chamomile tea bags in most

any store. Bulk chamomile can be bought cheaply in natural food markets and online. As always, I suggest choosing organic because it limits added chemicals and gives you a fresher product. 1-3 cups per day is the standard dose.

SALVE
For external inflammatory issues, such as eczema, rashes, sunburns and general itchiness or soreness, a salve with chamomile offers relief. The salve can be applied liberally to wounds or massaged onto sore body parts.

Recipe: Use the St. John's Wort Salve recipe in Chapter 1, only substitute an equal amount of chamomile for the St. John's Wort.

Chapter 3
Saw Palmetto and Vitex
His & Hers Hormonal
Balancing

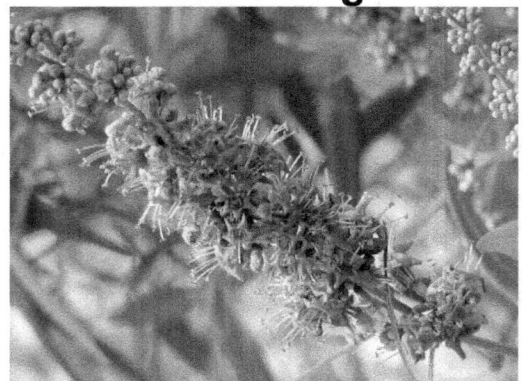

Vitex – photo credit: Stan Shebs

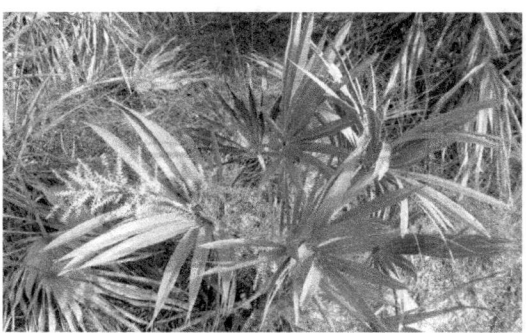

Saw Palmetto – photo credit: By Homer Edward Price

It's no wonder that our hormones are out of balance. Between a food supply laden with hormone disruptors, our lack of sleep and our stressful lifestyles, it's amazing that our endocrine system is working at all. The most common way to treat hormonal imbalance is with artificial hormone mimickers that often produce undesirable side effects. Herbal products are available for men and women to gently regulate hormones and bring the reproductive system back into place. Because these herbs do not grow in my region and I do not have the experience wildcrafting them, I am suggesting supplements of these wild or organically cultivated plants in the form of capsules and tinctures.

His: Saw Palmetto
Native to North America and commonly found in the southeastern states in sandy coastal areas and forest floors, this palm-like wild plant has been shown in studies to inhibit the production of the enzyme 5-alpha reductase. This action leads to the balancing of testosterone levels, which then has an overall positive impact in cases of sexual dysfunction.

Supplementing with Saw Palmetto has helped in cases of numerous male problems including loss of libido, prostate enlargement and male pattern hair loss. 320 mgs per day, either at one time or twice daily, in capsule form, for up to six months is the standard dose. When buying the supplement, look for labels that list the product at 85%-95% fatty acids and sterols, since it is these properties of the plant that produce the enzyme-inhibiting action.

WARNING: Saw Palmetto may have interactions with other drugs. Be sure to consult your healthcare practitioner before use.

Hers: Vitex

Vitex, with its large violet flowers, may remind some people of a lilac bush. Commonly known as Chasteberry, this tree-like herb originated in China and has been cultivated and spreading in the wild across the southern U.S. since the 17th century. Because of its overall effects on all stages of a woman's reproductive life, Vitex is known as the ultimate hormonal tonic for females.

Vitex acts specifically on the pituitary gland (the "Master Gland"), which in turn normalizes the production of luteinizing hormone, which regulates menstrual cycles. Because of its naturally balancing effects on estrogen and progesterone levels, Vitex promotes female reproductive health. Those supplementing with Vitex have shown alleviated PMS symptoms, increased fertility, normalized menstrual cycles, less bleeding, and relief from menopausal symptoms like hot flashes and depression.

16 ml of Vitex tincture per day for up to 18 months is the standard recommendation.

WARNING: Because there are so many naturally occurring hormones involved during pregnancy, Vitex is not recommended during this time.

Chapter 4
Milk Thistle
For Toxic Overload

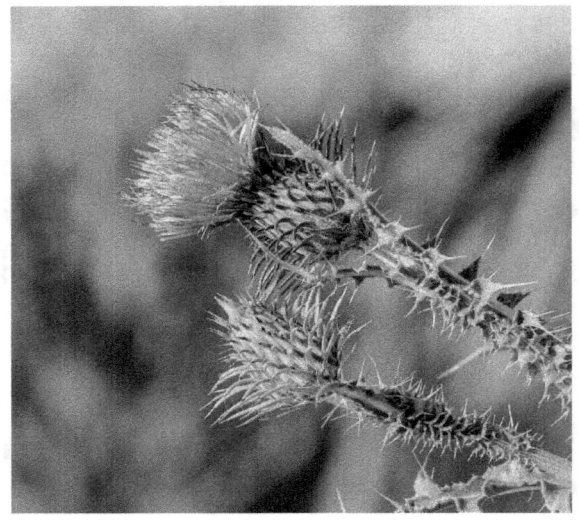

Do you remember those thorny, bristly flowers that Eeyore was always eating in Winnie the Pooh stories? The same purple plant that graces the cover of this book and was enjoyed as a meal by a melancholy donkey is the exact herb you want for optimal liver health.

The liver is our detoxification center. It filters the blood while removing toxins and metabolizing drugs and chemicals. If you think about the current lifestyle in western societies, it's easy to see that our livers are extremely overtaxed. This is shown in the preponderance of liver diseases like Hepatitis, Fatty Liver Disease, Cirrhosis, Acetaminophen Toxicity, Jaundice and Liver Cancer.

The active ingredient in Milk Thistle is Silymarin, which stabilizes the liver cell membranes and stimulates protein synthesis, which speeds up the liver regeneration process. It has also been shown to block harmful toxins from entering the liver's cells while improving the removal of these toxic chemicals.

While the stalks of the Milk Thistle plant can be peeled (using gloves) and eaten like celery, it is the seeds that contain the concentrated amounts of Silymarin that are so beneficial to your liver.

How To Use Milk Thistle

Only a hardcore forager would harvest milk thistle seeds for daily use. To do this you first enter the thistle patch wearing sturdy clothes and gloves and cut the thistles just under the bulbs in late summer. Dry them by placing the bulbs whole in a paper bag with a few air holes for several weeks. They are dried when the white, feathery down of the flower is light and fluffy. Pull out the down and you will see the seed, shaped like a date, stuck at the end. Separate the seeds from the down with your fingers and store in airtight jar. Grind seeds in a coffee grinder and add a teaspoon of the powder to your oatmeal or any recipe or smoothie. If you have the opportunity to wildcraft this herb, drying it and using daily or encapsulating yourself will save you money and give you a fresher product, but it does entail considerable work.

For those looking for a simpler way to optimize liver health, I would suggest starting with 200 mg capsules of the seed 1-3 times daily for up to 12 months. Since when taking Milk Thistle you are treating liver disorders, I highly recommend choosing the organic or locally sourced herbs.

Whether you are harvesting your own Milk Thistle or buying it, you can rest assured knowing that there are no identified negative side effects of this supplement.

Chapter 5
Eyebright
For Eye Strain

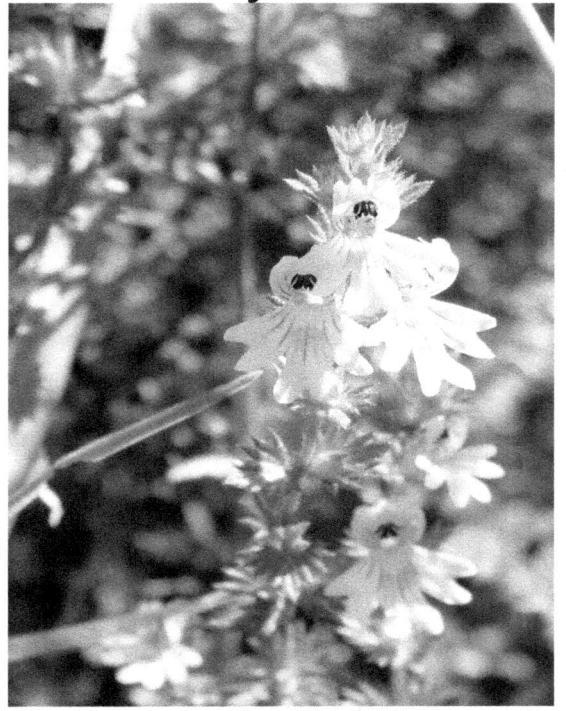

The other night, I took a break from writing and went for a walk. It was dark, but the moon was bright giving me the light I needed to see my way up the road and back. When I returned I could see a few lights on in the house, but what really stood out was my laptop that I had left open; it's bright white light standing out. I thought, "*man*, I stare at that light for hours at a time!" No wonder my eyes feel tired so often.

Many people do this for eight or more hours every day. When we are viewing the screens of our devices, we blink less than normal which can cause dryness and soreness. The intense focus can also be the root of headaches and other eye related symptoms. Relief can be achieved by taking frequent 'eye breaks' which involve looking at something in the distance every twenty minutes or so (there are even apps to remind you!), and making sure your screen is just below eye level. But the reality is many of us are spending a lot of time focusing intently on electronic devices and straining our eyes.

Symptoms of eye strain range from dry, sore, or itchy eyes, to headaches, light sensitivity and blurred vision. Mother Nature in her infinite wisdom has provided us with a wild herb that works directly to reduce the discomforts of eye strain and many other eye issues. Eyebright, a tiny flowered, weedy looking herb found wild in Europe, Asia and North America can be used to treat all eye disorders.

Eyebright's tannin content, which acts as an astringent, and its anti-inflammatory and antibacterial properties, combine to make the perfect eye wash. Its 3 major antioxidant vitamins bring in eye-specific support as well: Vitamin C, in conjunction with Eyebright's high content of Quercetin, assists in reducing swelled and runny eyes; Vitamin E has been shown to help improve visual sharpness; and Vitamin A protects the cornea and prevents dry eyes.

Eyebright is the perfect solution for eyestrain symptoms, but it can also be used for many other eye disorders including conjunctivitis and itchy or runny eyes caused by allergies. Traditionally it has been used to improve memory and treat vertigo and epilepsy.

Harvesting and drying Eyebright is easy. The high tannin content makes it a fast-drying herb. Simply cut the flowering tops of the plant and dry for a day or two in an oven with just the pilot light on, or in an airy spot out of the sun for several days. The dried herb will have retained its colors, though the flowers will have diminished considerably in size.

How To Use Eyebright

How to make an eye bath:
Boil 2 cups of water and pour over 1 cup of dried or fresh herb and let sit for 20 minutes or more. Strain well using cheesecloth or an unbleached coffee filter, store in a sterile glass jar (just dip in the boiling water before adding the herbs and let stand, open side up), cool, lid tightly and place in refrigerator for up to a week. When you wash your face in the morning or evening, use a sterile eyecup or other small sterile container to 'wash' your eyes with this herbal extract. If you are experiencing a painful eye condition, it is better to warm the eye bath liquid slightly before use. You can also dip cotton balls in the solution and press one on each eye (with lid closed) as a compress.

Eyebright Tea:
Using the same method for making an eye bath, simply drink the tea for relief

of eye symptoms due to eyestrain, colds and allergies.

Chapter 6
Melissa (Lemon Balm)
For Cold Sores and Herpes
Simplex

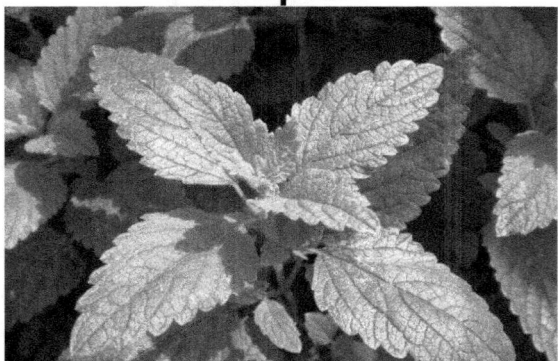

Otherwise known as Lemon Balm, Melissa Officinalis is well known for its direct antiviral effects on herpes viruses. While no cure for Herpes has been identified, Melissa provides a potent remedy for use against symptoms of the two major types of herpes viruses: Herpes Simplex 1 which usually manifests in cold sores; and Herpes Simplex 2 which causes genital herpes and is currently a worldwide problem with over 400,000,000 people currently living with this condition. Both types can result in painful sores, are highly contagious orally and sexually, and can even be passed from a pregnant mother to her unborn child.

Amazingly, using Melissa has been shown repeatedly to cut the time that herpes patients suffer from sores *in half*. In numerous other studies Melissa exhibited its use in preventing Herpes outbreaks. People who have used Melissa on painful cold sores and herpes blisters have noticed relief in as little as five minutes! Here are just a few of the numerous medicinal properties contained in Lemon Balm that work directly on this condition:

1. Eugenol - This antibacterial component can help reduce secondary infections and spreading while also acting as a nerve soother. Herpes symptoms can worsen in stressful situations and having this nerve toner helps to allay the effects.

2. Terpenes - Found in the essential oil of Melissa, terpenes soothe painful nerve tissues, helping to reduce the pain and discomfort of the sores and ulcers.

3. Tannins - Tannins inhibit the herpes virus' ability to be absorbed by non-affected cells, thus making Melissa a powerful antiviral.

How to Use Melissa

*Note: All the preparations listed below are effective strategies in dealing with Herpes viruses. You can use one or more at one time.

1. Essential Oil in a Natural Balm
Warm 5 parts coconut oil (which is also antiviral) and 1 part beeswax (or candelilla wax if vegan) until melted. Cool slightly and stir in 10-30 drops of Melissa pure essential oil, depending on how large a batch you are making. Pour into a glass container and put the lid on once completely cooled. Depending on the climate where you live, if you want the balm to be harder, add a bit more wax. If you need it to be softer, add a bit more coconut oil. Apply directly to sores, being sure to wash hands before and after use. *HINT*: If you have a salve or balm already that you bought or made and you want to add Melissa Essential Oil, simply melt it down in a pan (never boiling), pour back into its container, add

the essential oil, stir with a toothpick and let it harden back up.

2. Water Extract/Tea used externally
Pour 2 cups of boiling water over 1 cup of dried Melissa herb and steep for 20 minutes or more, Strain, cool and then dip a cotton ball in the liquid and apply directly to sores. Refrigerate and use for up to a week. No double dipping!

3. Water Extract/tea used internally
Same method as above in #2 except drink the tea, up to 3 cups per day.

4. Alcohol or Glycerin Extract (Tinctures) Take 15-30 drops of the tincture 3 times per day until 2 days after all symptoms are gone. May be taken under the tongue, or mixed with water or juice. Alcoholic tinctures taste very strong and may be undesirable to non-drinkers. Though not quite as strong as the alcoholic extracts, glycerin tinctures can also provide a strong level of relief.

Chapter 7
Boswellia
For Asthma

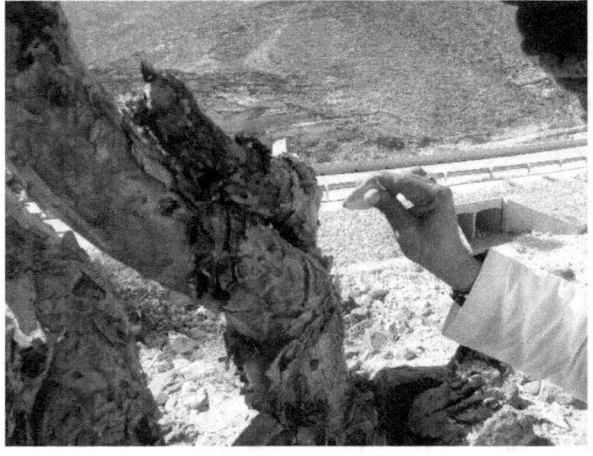

Photo Credit: By Mileli

In this chapter I had initially planned to highlight one of my favorite and most foraged herbs, Mullein, because of its respiratory healing properties. But while I was researching studies related to asthma I came across an herb that was repeatedly mentioned as showing improvements in asthmatic symptoms. Otherwise known as Indian Frankincense, Boswellia proved to be the best herb to be featured in this chapter about asthma.

Native to India, Northern Africa and the Arabian Peninsula, it's not an herb I have ever come across in my wanderings here in the Northeastern United States. For centuries, and still today, frankincense is used in religious ceremonies and its scent is believed to foster a heightened spirituality.

The gum resin from the Boswellia tree has been traditionally used for many ailments and has also been studied extensively for its beneficial actions in asthma cases. This resin, with its ability to affect all chronic inflammatory diseases, works especially well in decreasing asthma symptoms.

Boswellic Acid, found in the resin, inhibits the production of leukotrienes, which can trigger asthmatic bronchial contractions. Taking this powerful herb has been shown to reduce the overall severity of asthma attacks, and their frequency.

There are many different species of Boswellia and all have powerful anti-inflammatory effects, but the papyrifera species found in Somalia, Ethiopia, Oman and Yemen have tested as the most potent. To harvest this herb, you can simply break off the resin that has built up on the outside of the tree, or peel off the papery outer bark and make a cut in the inner bark to catch the flow of resin, harvesting it once it has hardened. If you live in an area where this tree grows, taking the resin that has already built up on the outside of the tree is the least invasive method of collection. The hardened resin can be then extracted using petroleum or ethanol, or using olive oil. Using and/or seeking out the oil based solutions when purchasing this supplement is most likely the healthiest option.

WARNING: Only people who are in healthy condition, other than the asthma, should consider taking Boswellia. It may cause a worsening of other disease symptoms (other than asthma) and can interact adversely with prescription medications. Pregnant woman should not take Boswellia. Check with your healthcare provider before taking Boswellia.

How to use Boswellia

Recommended dosage information listed on the supplement bottle should be noted. Usually, 300 mg three times per day for up to six weeks is the standard.

Chapter 8
Psyllium
For Type 2 Diabetes

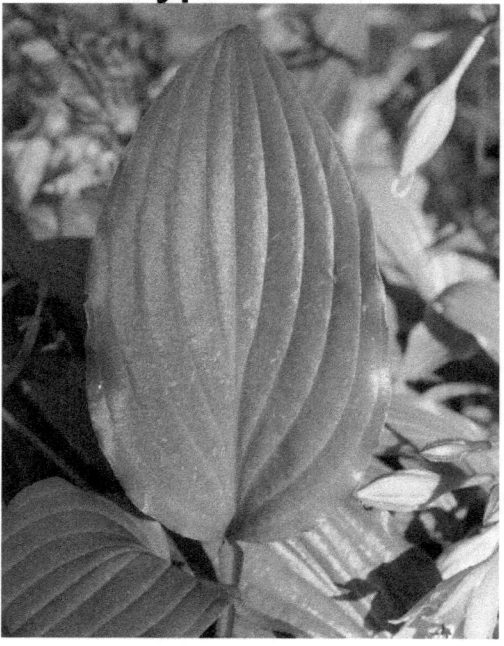

Currently in the United States, over 9% of our population has Type 2 Diabetes, a condition in which a person's blood sugar rises higher than normal due to insulin resistance or insufficient insulin production. Symptoms of this disease, such as frequent urination, increased hunger and fatigue can be reduced or eliminated in time with lifestyle changes (exercise and diet). Since Type 2 Diabetes can also lead to cardiovascular disease and stroke, it's smart to include a gentle, effective remedy while lifestyle issues are addressed and excess weight is lost.

Psyllium, the seed husk of herbs in the plantain family, makes the perfect natural treatment with its high content of soluble fiber. Tested extensively, it's been shown to cause major improvements in glucose values. Supplementing with Psyllium twice a day before lunch and dinner significantly reduces the fasting blood sugar levels and post-meal glucose levels as shown in human subjects in numerous studies. Overall, Psyllium is a safe, widely tolerated solution to improving blood sugar levels.

The Psyllium found online and in stores for sale as a supplement is most likely from the species Plantago Ovata grown commercially in Eastern Europe and Asia. A close relative, Plantago Major (or Broadleaf Plantain), though originating in the same areas as Ovata, now grows wild all over North America. The Psyllium is the outer covering of the seeds on the stalk of the plant.

The whole plant, including leaves and roots can be used medicinally, but the parts used for supplementing in Type 2 Diabetes are the ground seed husks. If you have Broadleaf Plantain growing in your yard like I do, you can easily see the seed husks growing straight up out of the leaves. While I was outside today, I ate a few of the seeds with the husks on. The seeds are extremely mucilaginous, or oily textured, and I found that when I ate the husks without the seeds, I liked the taste a lot better. But since they are so tiny, I think as a wildcrafter, if I wanted to enjoy the glucose stabilizing effects of the Psyllium, I would just eat them whole, as it would take a long time to separate the tiny seeds from the husks. They could certainly be dried and then later ground up with a coffee grinder and added to smoothies, soups or baked goods recipes.

WARNING: Psyllium may affect the potency of other laxatives, medications and supplements. It is advised to take it two hours before or after another remedy, natural or otherwise.

How to Use Psyllium

You can eat this herb raw as a daily herbal supplement as I described above, or take 5.5g of the powdered seed husk twice a day before lunch and dinner. Always mix powdered Psyllium in with a large glass of water to dilute the mucilage.

Chapter 9
Yellow Dock
For Skin Problems

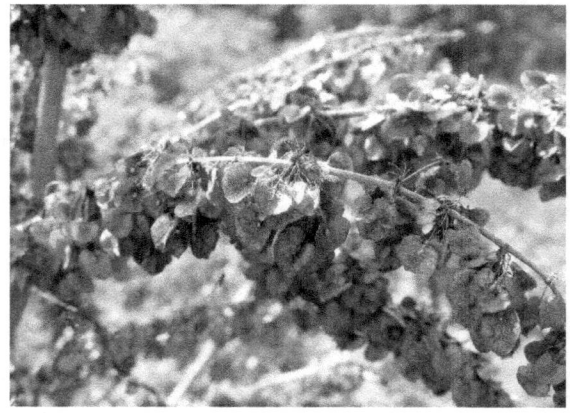

One of the most iron dense plants on earth, Yellow Dock represents a foraged medicinal herb that is easily found and harvested, and that works to eliminate toxins from the blood in support of the skin.

In particular, the root of Yellow Dock contains high amounts of anthraquinone, a plant constituent that stimulates bile production and activates the nerve center in the intestine. This stimulation of the stomach muscles leads to the mobilization of congested blood. Overall this herb can have profound effects on the skin through its blood cleansing powers.

For the 30 million plus eczema sufferers in the U.S. alone, supplementing with Yellow Dock can detoxify the skin from the inside out and reduce eczema symptoms. Eating a wholesome diet, using natural fibers that allow skin to breathe, and eliminating common food triggers like wheat, eggs and dairy has been shown to reduce or eliminate outbreaks. In fact, I have been completely eczema free since giving up dairy and gluten products. Allergens may also be to blame as well as microbes, extreme temperatures and chemical irritants in body care products. But if eczema is severe or you are not able to pinpoint the cause, I highly recommend Yellow Dock supplementation.

This wild herb is also effective in cases of acne, psoriasis and other skin rashes. Most practitioners will tell you that eczema has no known external cause. Thus it makes sense to treat this disease internally instead of applying topical treatments.

To find Yellow Dock it's easiest to identify the plant in the fall, when the tall seed stock turns a rich, earthy brown and stands in contrast to the waning colors of the grasses and fields where it lives. In the spring, copious green leaves grow and can be used in many recipes but they are not a sustenance food because of their high oxalic acid content (like spinach, you would not eat this every day). The stalks can be eaten as well but early spring and summer are when they are most tender.

Of all the parts of Yellow Dock, the roots by far contain the highest level of detoxification power. They can be harvested, sliced and dried for future use in a tea, or tinctured fresh or dried for long-term storage and use. See my YouTube channel, Boondocks Botanicals, for two videos about harvesting and using Yellowdock.

How To Use Yellow Dock - Tincture Making

Secure quality hooch

If you can get locally made alcohol and/or organic hooch, I would definitely use that. In Maine we are blessed with abundant potatoes and I can buy locally made vodka. Everclear (grain alcohol) can also be used. For some, the taste of the alcohol is too strong or otherwise undesirable. In these cases glycerin or apple cider vinegar can be used to make the tincture, but they do not draw out the same amount of plant properties that alcohol will. However, either of these extraction methods would still make a great second choice. I have a friend who has also used local apple brandy, which makes for a nicer tasting tincture, with slightly less potency than stronger alcoholic products.

Once you have secured the hooch, simply use a glass jar, fill ⅔ full with dried herb, and cover to fill with alcohol or other chosen menstruum. A tincture will be ready to go after a few weeks and the herbs can be strained out. What's left is your tincture. Many herbalists, including me, leave the herbs for longer, some for months or years. I usually will leave the herbs in for at least 4-5 weeks.

Storing the tinctures in dark glass will prolong their potency, though alcohol tinctures in general have a pretty long shelf life.

Tincture Dosing

For eczema and other skin disorders, take 15-30 drops of the tincture under the tongue (as long as you can, then swallow), twice daily until symptoms improve, for up to six months.

How to Use Yellow Dock - Making a Tea

Using dried slivers, or crushed or ground Yellow Dock root, add 3 teaspoons of the herb to 2 cups of boiling water, simmer on low for 20 minutes, strain and drink. 1-3 cups per day is recommended.

Chapter 10
Motherwort
For Heart Disease

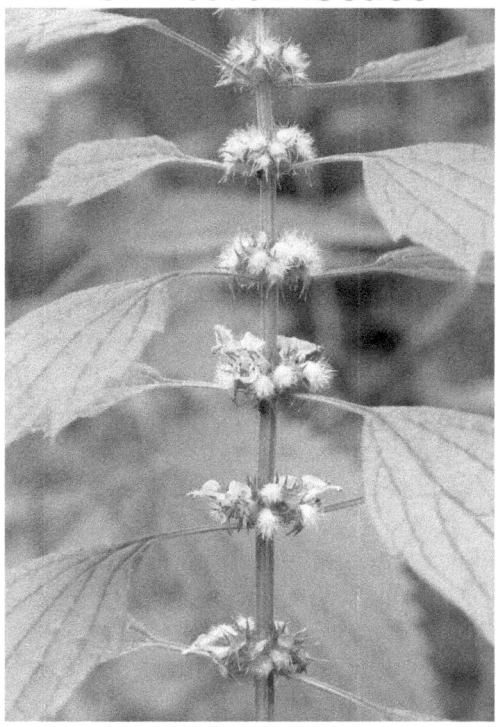

If ever there was a wild herb for today's problems, I think Motherwort would be it. The way this plant acts on the nervous system and the cardiovascular system in tandem creates a natural remedy for the stresses of modern life that take their toll on our bodies.

The Latin name for this herb, Leonurus Cardiaca, is derived from the Greek words lion tail and heart. A quick look at the herb and you can see the similarity of the leaves to a lion's tail. The second part of the name directly reflects this herb's influence on the heart. Together, lionhearted is exactly what this plant resembles in its effects on humans. The Motherwort nickname came from its widespread traditional use for women in labor to relieve their tension. A member of the mint family, Motherwort is Native to Europe and Asia, but has become naturalized throughout North America.

While many people consider this plant to be primarily a woman's herb because of its long history of use relating to the female reproductive system, Motherwort offers modern humanity a gentle way to reduce stress and the ill health effects caused by the resulting strain.

Motherwort is a hypotensive herb, which means it has the power to lower blood pressure and reduce heart palpitations brought on by tension and anxiety. An all around cardiac tonic, this herb calms the excess energy throughout the nervous system and heart, decreases clotting and blood fat levels, and is a mild sedative and diuretic, directly aiding the lowering of blood pressure and reducing stress. Motherwort traditionally has been used to calm nervous complaints, ease insomnia and act as a heart tonic in all circulation disorders.

How does Motherwort do all this? The answer lies mainly in the alkaloid 'leonurine' which is a gentle vasodilator, an antioxidant and an anti-spasmodic. This plant constituent relaxes the smooth muscular tissues of the heart. Motherwort calms and tones the distressed heart.

How to Use Motherwort

Motherwort Tea
To make a cup of Motherwort tea, simply pour a cup of boiling water over 2-3 teaspoons of the dried herb, cover and wait 15 minutes, then drink. 1-3 cups per day would be the standard dose.

Motherwort Tincture

Follow the instructions for tincture making in Chapter 9, only using Motherwort as the herb. Taking 5-10 drops under the tongue 2-3 times per day is recommended.

Conclusion:
Embracing a Natural Choice

We are so lucky to have the exact plants growing on our planet that can help us with the health problems we have created in modern life. By having an attitude that embraces the abundance that nature provides, and by avoiding the unnecessary depletion of wildlife, we are only helping ourselves build better lives.

Foraging for wild medicinal herbs teaches us that we have the power within ourselves to heal. This is a lesson I plan to continually study as I see the rampant deterioration of health in humans today. It is my hope to make foraging for wild herbs as mainstream as taking an aspirin for a headache. It is my goal to see the world as a place where people look to the root of their health problems so they may enjoy a better life, brought to them by a little wellness from the wild.

Thank you reading. I would love to hear your input so please be sure to leave a review at Amazon.com, look for Mary Thibodeau, and please do not hesitate to mention herbs or health issues you would like to see addressed in my upcoming books.